Spontaneous

REMISSION

A mind-blowing true story,
fostering hope

ANNE W. WHEELER

HERE I AM
PUBLISHING, LLC

Printed in the United States of America.
ISBN (Hardback): 978-1-958032-30-5
ISBN (Paperback): 978-1-958032-32-9
This book is a work of non-fiction.

Copyright © 2025 by Anne W. Wheeler

Scripture quotations marked NIV are taken from the Holy Bible, New International Version ®, NIV ®. Copyright © 1973, 1978, 1984, 2011 by Biblica, Inc.™ Used by permission of Zondervan. All rights reserved worldwide. www.zondervan.com The "NIV" and "New International Version" are trademarks registered in the United States Patent and Trademark Office by Biblica, Inc.™

Scripture quotations are from the ESV® Bible (The Holy Bible, English Standard Version®), copyright © 2001 by Crossway, a publishing ministry of Good News Publishers. Used by permission. All rights reserved."

Permissions have been obtained from those in the story. All rights reserved. No part of this book may be used or reproduced by any means, graphic, electronic, or mechanical, including photocopying, recording, taping, or by any information storage retrieval system without the written permission of the publisher except in the case of brief quotations embodied in critical articles and reviews.

Graphic Artist Jennifer Gunn
Sandi Huddleston-Edwards, Publisher
Published by Here I Am Publishing, LLC
780 Monterrosa Drive
Myrtle Beach, South Carolina 29572

Dedication

During my journey, while deeply personal, I was never truly alone. This is a collective testament to the grace, power of faith, the resilience of the human spirit, and the enduring strength found in the love and support of those around us. It is dedicated to every soul touched by cancer and those who tirelessly fight alongside them. It is dedicated to everyone who has ever faced an insurmountable challenge, reminding them that even in the darkest of nights, there is always a light waiting to shine through.

May my book offer solace, hope, and a renewed belief in the boundless love of the divine.

- To my unwavering faith, which has carried me through the darkest waters and into the sunlit waves.
- To Bill, my family, and friends, whose love and support were my lifeline during times of immense fear and uncertainty.
- To the medical professionals who provided exceptional care and unwavering compassion, even when faced with the inexplicable.

Miracles are, and always were, one of God's many gifts.

Prologue

My journey began with a diagnosis that shattered my world: cancer. That unwelcome guest had invaded my life, filling my days with fear, uncertainty, and a deep sense of vulnerability.

The medical landscape was both overwhelming and often devoid of true hope in those early days. But amid the turmoil, something remarkable happened. My faith, previously a quiet background hum in my life, became my anchor. It was not a perfect faith; it was a wrestling, questioning, and evolving faith – messy, raw, and undeniably real.

This is not a story of unwavering piety but a story of a very human journey of faith, struggle, and miraculous healing. In the depths of despair, it was the unwavering belief in something greater than myself that kept me going. I offer this narrative, not as a testament to my spiritual perfection, but as a testament to the power of faith and prayer to sustain, to heal, and to lead even through utter bewilderment. Within these pages, you will find not only my story but an invitation to explore your own relationship with our Lord and the extraordinary strength you possess to overcome adversity.

My prayer is that my experiences will bring hope, encouragement, and a renewed sense of possibilities to those traversing similar paths.

Table of Contents

Introduction

The unexpected can strike at any moment,
often without warning.

In November 2022, I received the life-altering news of a cancer diagnosis. The impact was immediate, profound, and utterly terrifying. The initial wave of fear and uncertainty threatened to engulf me. Yet, even during the darkest hours, a quiet strength emerged from within. My faith, a constant companion throughout my childhood and early parental years, had faltered for many years. But I had renewed my faith recently (2019 to present), and it became my unwavering anchor, guiding me through the storm.

In October 2024, I faced another cancer diagnosis, an experience that once again tested the limits of my faith. The unexpected resolution of this second diagnosis left not only medical professionals and all of us baffled, but it strengthened my belief in the power of divine intervention. This is not merely a tale of miraculous healings; it is a raw and honest account of a personal relationship with God, intertwined with the very real struggles, anxieties, and uncertainties that accompany such a journey. It is a story of human vulnerability and the transformative power of faith, hope, and unwavering belief.

CHAPTER 1

The Shattering News and Initial Reactions

He is not afraid of bad news;
his heart is firm, trusting in the Lord.
—Psalm 112.7 (ESV)

The year 2022 will be a historically bad year for my health record book. From knee surgery and recovery; to Covid-19 illness; to shoulder injury, shoulder surgery, and shoulder physical therapy; and with my five-year follow-up colonoscopy; but the worst was yet to come.

My colonoscopy was scheduled for late September, and all the preparation paperwork was handed to me at the pre-surgery doctor meeting. I requested an endoscopy at the same time, as I was experiencing discomfort while eating in the prior months. So, I made a quick trip to the pharmacy to purchase all the items needed to clean out my system and to be consumed starting the day before the colonoscopy and endoscopy.

The preparation fluids and fasting began, and as the late evening came, I started feeling a slight headache, so I went to bed. The headache became so severe by 2 a.m., I woke up my partner, Bill, to ask for his help. My head felt like it was going to explode. He immediately took my blood pressure twice in both arms, and the look on his face told me all I needed to know. He immediately called for an ambulance to take me to the hospital. My blood pressure was at stroke level.

The ensuing three days in the hospital were filled with a barrage of tests and different drugs to help lower my blood pressure but to no avail. Just being in the hospital made my blood pressure rise. The brain MRI, heart stress test, blood tests, and other tests showed nothing was wrong. I had repeatedly told many doctors and nurses what seemed like a hundred times about prepping for my colonoscopy and endoscopy, yet no one was able to figure out why my normal blood pressure went so dangerously high and why it was not coming down.

On the third day, my blood pressure came down enough for them to release me. I was happy to be able to go home and sleep in my bed without being poked, prodded, and given blood pressure checks all night long. I knew I would be able to rest at home. I was told to follow up with my family doctor.

October was a blur after that stress-filled stay in the hospital. Thankfully, I obtained an appointment with my family doctor within ten days of my hospital stay. I had a fresh set of ears to hear the details of what happened, and my doctor recommended I just skip the colonoscopy and get an endoscopy. He felt the prep drugs set off something in my stomach, which is what sent my blood pressure souring. He wanted to rule out the big "C" (Cancer) as its cause. He explained that when your body is injured, your blood pressure rises as your body is trying to heal the injury.

Within a week, an endoscopy was performed, and a small area in my stomach, which did not look normal, was biopsied. I was told the results would be available within seven–ten days. Those were the longest days of my life, waiting to hear the results.

My doctor called and spoke in a calm voice; he did not like the results and wanted to double-check the lab results at MUSC (The Medical University of South Carolina). In the meantime, I checked my patient portal and saw the results. I started to research the results through *Google*. I did not really grasp what I read but realized why my doctor wanted to double check it. I felt it was best to wait for confirmation. Another seven to ten days of an agonizing wait for results.

The world tilted on its axis that early November afternoon. The GI (gastroenterologist) doctor's words, precise and clinical, hung in the air like shards of glass, each syllable a tiny, agonizing cut.

"Signet Ring Adenocarcinoma Stomach Cancer," was confirmed again by the second pathology report at MUSC, he'd said, with a voice devoid of the usual bedside manner. It was now replaced by a stark, unvarnished reality. The phrase echoed in my ears, a relentless drumbeat of fear and disbelief. My carefully constructed life, brimming with December 28 travel plans to Israel and the hope of walking where Jesus walked, crumbled before me like a sandcastle in a storm.

The news felt surreal, a cruel twist in a script I hadn't written and a plotline I never imagined. How could this be happening to *me*? I was a mostly healthy, athletic, active, woman of faith who regularly attended church. I was someone who felt deeply connected to God's love and grace. Surely, this was a mistake, a cruel joke.

But the pathology report wasn't a joke. I immediately opened *Google* to see what I was dealing with. I have always researched topics of concern or interest, and the images and text of this type of cancer on the screen were stark and undeniable: a malignant growth, a predator quietly consuming a part of me.

My cancer was known to be the deadliest stomach cancer if not detected early. This cancer insidiously grows in the multiple linings of your stomach and can quickly find its way out to other organs. The initial shock gave way to a wave of overwhelming grief. Tears streamed down my face, hot and unstoppable as the enormity of the situation washed over me. I had lost my namesake, my Aunt Anne, to stomach cancer many years earlier.

Surely, there are much better survival rates or cures by now. My thoughts of my now grown children losing their mom after having lost their dad to lung cancer nine years prior just crushed my heart. It felt as if the ground had fallen away, leaving me suspended in a void of fear and uncertainty.

My partner, Bill, who was new in my life at the beginning of 2021, became my pillar of strength. Early on, he showed me his strong character and his love and willingness to take care of me no matter what. He wanted to marry me, but I struggled with trust, due to a prior failed relationship that broke my heart like a delicate vase.

Now, this wonderful man, who quietly sat with me through this, never let me see his own fears of loss; instead, he showed me strength. He had lost his wife, the mother of his children, to breast cancer at a young age. At this point, his usual boisterous energy was subdued and replaced by a quiet strength that anchored me in the storm. He had happily renewed his faith when we became a couple, turning into a rock-solid belief in God's plan, even amid life's challenges. But this felt different. This was a challenge of a magnitude I had never encountered. ***How could we navigate this together when our future seemed so irrevocably altered?***

The days that followed were a blur of calls for appointments, consultations, and medical jargon. I spent hours online, researching the disease, reading about survival rates, reading success stories, and reading horrifying statistics. It was a treacherous path, an endless loop of hope and despair. The Internet, meant to offer information and support, instead created a labyrinth of anxiety. Regardless of that, I have always believed that knowledge is power. Instead, I decided that God had this. He is the ultimate healer. I leaned into prayer.

The next day I was scheduled to attend my monthly Christian Ladies' LIFE luncheon. It is a wonderful and supportive group of ladies. I struggled with my decision to attend or whether I should tell anyone for fear I would not be able to keep my composure. My extremely sensitive nature leads me to cry easily. I didn't want to show my fear and anxiety, but I soon found that my faith and these loving Christian ladies would help me get through it. When I told the leading ladies of our group about my diagnosis, they made a special point to ask for prayers from the forty ladies in attendance. Some laid hands directly on me. I felt the love of Jesus giving me strength, and I am forever grateful to all those ladies who shared their compassion and faith with me. Their faith and mine filled me with great strength and love.

By mid-November, my GI doctor referred me to an oncologist close by, and I arrived at a wonderful caring cancer center. My oncologist was kind, listened intently, and made recommendations to find out my cancer stage. Through the blood tests, the CT scans, and MRI PET scan, we determined that I was at an early stage 1, and it hadn't spread elsewhere. I drew a big sigh of relief for the time being. The most important part of cancer is knowing what kind, how much invasion, and how to remove it expeditiously.

I knew from my first husband's cancer diagnosis that the PET scan would only determine if the cancer had spread. I was told that the stomach needed to be reviewed from the inside, and the PET scan would not be able to see the cancer in my stomach. I needed to have a GI oncologist do an endoscopy with ultrasound and biopsies. I was referred to a GI oncology group in Conway, not too far from home.

Hurry up and wait! I was warned by others who have lived through the cancer journey that waiting for answers is as bad as the cancer diagnosis. The GI oncologist they referred was booked for months. I waited until Friday to call the GI oncologist group again, asking if there were any cancellations for that specific doctor. Time is so important. The stress of waiting consumes you.

Low and behold, there was a new GI oncologist that had just moved to the area, and one of his few new patients had cancelled, and I was given the endoscopy surgery appointment the following Tuesday morning. Divine intervention? I believe it was. I was so thankful to find a very highly qualified GI oncologist to do an ultrasound, laparoscopically review of my stomach, and take more biopsies to get an exact picture of what I was dealing with.

Nearly two months had passed since the initial endoscopy and diagnosis in early October. It seemed like a year. The drive to Conway was a mix of quiet and nervous discussion about what was to come. We both tried to show optimism about the diagnosis of stage 1 cancer, but this endoscopy would tell us whether chemo or radiation would be in the picture and if our trip to Israel would be attainable. We quietly prayed.

The weight of the diagnosis and what was to come pressed heavily on my partner, Bill. His love and support were my lifeline, but I could see the worry etched on his face, the unspoken questions in his eyes. He tried to offer comfort, but I knew his own heart was burdened with his anxiety for me. I wanted to shield him from the anxiety, but how could I? How could I hide the turmoil within me? He had lost his wife to cancer and did his best to hide his own anxiety to give me strength.

"For I know the plans I have for you,"
declares the Lord, "plans to prosper you and not
to harm you, plans to give you hope and a future."
—Jeremiah 29:11 (NIV)

CHAPTER 2

Early Prayers and Spiritual Practices

*But when Jesus heard it he said, "This illness does not
lead to death. It is for the glory of God, so that
the Son of God may be glorified through it."*
—John 11:4 (ESV)

T he sterile scent of the surgery preparation room still clung to my clothes, a phantom smell that lingered even after I had left its confines. The fear, however, remained a constant companion, a shadow clinging to the edges of my consciousness. The friendly nurses completed their many questions, the fluid line was inserted into my tiny veins, and the GI oncology surgeon entered the room to introduce himself and give me a run-down of what he was going to do. His professional, yet comfortable, nature was a welcome feeling.

He answered our many questions with great patience and knowledge. After we asked our final question, the answer threw us both for a loop. If the cancer's depth is to the outer layer and is widespread, the oncologist's recommendation is to remove the stomach. Bill and I glanced at each other with wide eyes of shock.

The surgeon's words replayed on a loop in my mind, each repetition sharpening the blade of dread, as I was wheeled into surgery. But even as the fear gnawed at me, something else stirred within – a deep, instinctive turning toward faith. It was not a conscious decision, not initially; it was more of a reflex, an ingrained response to crisis. Bill admitted to me later he was a nervous wreck while he waited for me to come out of surgery and prayed for God's merciful hand to heal me, to give me grace.

I was groggy when I awoke from surgery, but I was happy to see the nurses and Bill. The surgeon came in to give us his findings. He said that he had taken thirty-six biopsies in a mapped format in my stomach. I had some damage from acid reflux, but there was not anything that he saw that had him overly concerned. The pathology results would take about seven to ten days to return.

Again, hurry up and wait! Others, who had been through a cancer scenario had warned me about waiting anxiety. It was true. It was like hanging from a frayed rope over a deep chasm, praying someone would come along and save me. I spent those days keeping busy with friends and praying for good news. Sleepless nights affected Bill and me, making us edgy, and the days were just as long. We prayed together and alone. We held hands tightly while watching *The Chosen*, Jesus' story and talking about our hope to fulfill our plans to travel to Israel.

My upbringing had been steeped in the Catholic faith. I had fallen away from the Catholic church in my thirties. Now, in my late fifties, I fell in love with the church I found in 2019. I was re-baptized in the Baptist faith in 2021. Church was not just a Sunday ritual; it became the heart of my new relationship with God, a place of solace, community, and unwavering belief.

I was at a friend's birthday dinner celebration when my cell phone rang. It was my GI oncologist. I left the table, heart pounding, waiting to hear the diagnosis. As I stood outside the restaurant and then paced back and forth, the words I heard made me jump up and down. None of the thirty-six biopsies showed any cancer. I could not believe my ears! How could this be? Divine intervention? I believed it was.

I was told the ultrasound did not show anything either. I still could not believe it and verified it again by asking, "Is it possible that the original biopsy samples got all the cancer?" He said he believed so; however, I would need to have an endoscopy every three months for a year and then every six months for the next following two to three years. I ran into the restaurant with happy tears filling my eyes. All my friends were so excited for me. Bill was just as excited when I called him a brief time later.

God came through to give Bill and me a new lease on life. I could hear the relief in his voice and could not wait to hold him in my arms. We both gave praise to God and continue to do so. With each follow-up appointment, we held our breath and prayed.

We continued to thank God for His miracle, and our faith strengthened. We continued to follow His word through our Bible studies. We invited many friends to join us at our church, and we are proud to say we have brought many who loved it just as much as we did. The pastors and staff are so welcoming and helpful.

The initial shock of the diagnosis had created a period of intense introspection. I found myself examining my life, not with judgment, but with a renewed sense of perspective. The challenges I faced brought into sharp focus the things that truly mattered: faith, family, and the importance of cherishing every moment. The cancer, in its horrific way, had become a catalyst for spiritual growth for both Bill and me. **Israel, here we come!**

"The cords of death entangled me, the anguish of the grave came over me; I was overcome by distress and sorrow."
Psalm 116:3 (NIV)

CHAPTER 3

Miracles Never Cease

Now faith is the assurance of things hoped for,
the conviction of things not seen.
—Hebrews 11:1 (ESV)

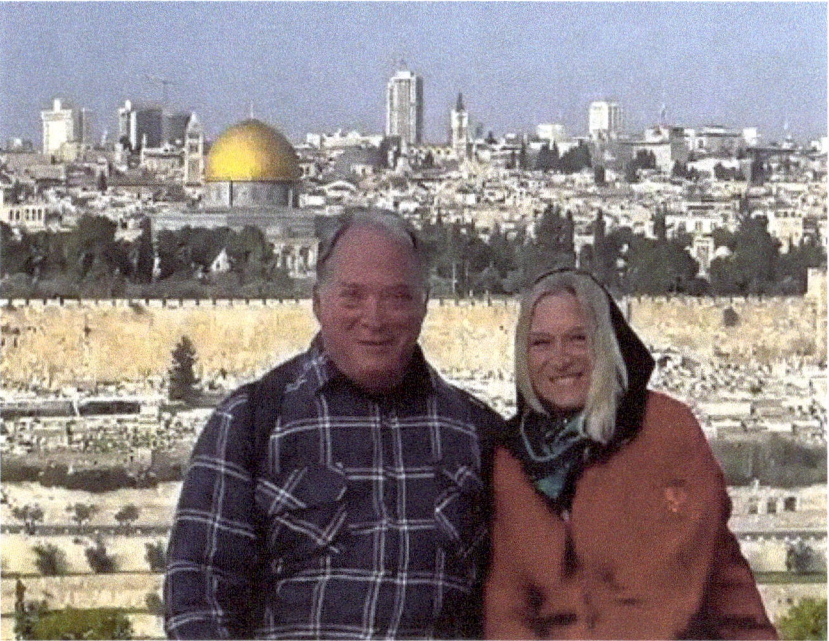

We were so excited to be able to join thirty-five of our faith-filled church community to Israel. It just did not seem real after what had transpired with my cancer diagnosis and with only two weeks to spare to potentially cancel our reservation. God wanted us to share in this special trip, and we were so thankful we were going.

Israel was filled with amazing history, and our tour was highlighted by Jesus' life: where He lived, where He performed His many miracles, where He was born, and where He died and was buried. The stone rolled away from the tomb was still there. The Bible came to life! The stories and structures left behind became a spiritual awakening for Bill and me.

A highlight on our trip was the Jordan River, which was set up for people to be baptized without standing in mud. The complex also had bathrooms to shower and change into dry clothes. Bill had voiced his desire to be baptized again, as he was an infant when he was brought into the Episcopal faith. Now, he was ready to personally recommit his faith in God. I had done so at our church the prior year. But I was compelled by my miracle to give thanks and to renew my faith by being baptized in the Jordan River. I had been born again by His healing, giving me new life. What an amazing experience!

I learned to find gratitude in the smallest things – the warmth of the sun on my skin, the laughter with my friend groups, and the comforting presence of my *soon to be spouse*.

Yes, miracles never cease to happen. While we were in Israel, one of our stops was in Bethlehem at a boutique featuring hand carved olive wood items and jewelry. Bill requested I look at some rings. I was happy to oblige since I was looking at another counter of jewelry, earrings/necklace sets. He wanted to propose marriage with a ring that I would be proud to wear. Up to this point, I was hesitant to consider getting married again. After experiencing all the love and care Bill had bestowed upon me during so many health issues that year, I knew he was the kind of man I could trust to be there for me through thick and thin.

While glancing through different engagement rings, one caught my eye. It was a blue diamond surrounded by little white diamonds. I was mesmerized by its simple beauty, and it was just the right sized diamond and setting for my little hand. I had not seen a blue diamond in over thirty years. He purchased it for me, and I told him that whenever he felt the desire to ask me, he could do so.

Little did I know he was not going to wait to ask me over a romantic dinner when we returned home. He knelt on one knee the next morning at breakfast in front of most of our fellow travelers. I was so shocked and surprised; the happy tears streamed down my face, as I said, "Yes." He had told many people from our group the night before about his plan to ask me to marry him at breakfast, and they were ready to take pictures of our special moments. I was so surprised and excited; I hardly ate my breakfast. Bill had waited two years to hear me say "Yes."

I learned that faith is not the absence of doubt; it is the capacity to believe despite the doubt. It is the ability to hold onto hope even when hope seems lost. It is the unwavering trust that God's plan, even when incomprehensible, is good and loving. It is a journey, not a destination, and a continuous process of growth, learning, and trusting in the unseen.

As I shared my miracle with others, so many people were amazed. They all felt relieved for us. They listened intently, asked questions, and celebrated with us. The outpouring of curiosity made me tempted to author a book. Through one of the presentations at my ladies' LIFE group, I heard something that sparked a title. I entered it into my phone but did not use it. Why was I not compelled to write it at the time? Fear? Doubt about my ability to write? Not enough content? It was a miracle, we agreed, but where do I start?

Upon our return from our glorious trip to Israel, 2023 was filled with conversations of where and when in 2024 we would be married. We still had the follow up endoscopies and tests every three months, which were like being on a roller coaster: excitement for our impending marriage plans, fear the cancer may come back, and then happiness that all was okay. After each endoscopy that year, the GI oncologist would say to us, "If I didn't know why you were here, I wouldn't know why you are here."

Each endoscopy gave way to anxiety until we heard those words "the results were negative for cancer." We continuously prayed and thanked our Lord for His healing. We shared our story to bring hope to others.

Looking back, I see my journey as a transformative experience, a pilgrimage of faith and healing. It was a journey that took me to despair, but it also led me to an unprecedented level of spiritual intimacy with God. The miracles were not just the inexplicable recoveries; they were the small moments of hope, the quiet whispers of divine grace, the unwavering love and support of my community, and the profound spiritual awakening that transformed my life.

Through it all, I learned the power of faith, not as a magical cure-all, but as a source of strength, resilience, and unwavering hope in the face of adversity. My journey is a testament to the enduring power of faith, the remarkable capacity of the human spirit, and the boundless love of a compassionate God.

It is a story of hope, of healing, and of unwavering faith in the face of the unimaginable. And it is a story I share not to boast of my strength, but to offer encouragement and inspiration to others who find themselves on similar journeys. The path is arduous, the challenges immense, but the reward—a deepened connection with God and the strength to face any obstacle—is beyond measure.

CHAPTER 4

The Unexpected New Diagnosis

> *But he said, "What is impossible with man is possible with God."*
> *—Luke 18:27 (ESV)*

The initial euphoria of my miracle – the early diagnosis, initial biopsy removal of my cancer, and the feeling of having cheated death had faded. The memory of that triumphant moment and the tears of joy shared with Bill, my family, friends, and my faith community, now felt like a distant dream.

The following year, 2023, we decided to take a cruise trip to the Mexican Riviera, a beautiful trip down the Southern West Coast of California into the Baha of California, along the Pacific Ocean to several small-town ports. God's hand in the rock formations, the blue waters, and fun towns was breathtaking. It was here that we decided to buy our wedding bands. Our hearts were filled with happiness. My continued testing results also showed that I truly was cured of that ugly cancer, and all the stress began to subside. We were focused through 2023 and the beginning of 2024 on our wedding plans and getting back to normalcy.

We celebrated our wedding on June 1, 2024, followed by a visit to California to share my grandson's fifth birthday and to start our honeymoon with a land and sea adventure in Alaska. Even though a fire in Denali and then rain dampened our trip, what I could see of Alaska was magnificent. It was the most beautiful trip we've enjoyed.

Upon our return, life went back to normal until I severely injured my left foot and had to wear a boot for six weeks and then a wrap for another six. Little did I know that this turn of events would start an avalanche of illness and fears.

It was October, and my annual allergies started to get the best of me. I had visited the doctor on an early October morning, because I was running a fever and had chest congestion for a couple of days. Throughout the day, I ran errands, but by midafternoon, my left leg became unbearably painful.

When I returned home, I discovered that my left leg, from thigh to toe, had blown up like a balloon. I immediately knew what it was: a blood clot!

Bill rushed me to the hospital, and they reacted quickly to send me into an emergency room. An ultrasound determined that there was extraordinarily little blood circulating down my leg, and they were not sure where the blockage was. Shortly after that, a CT scan with contrast was performed.

After an hour later, several doctors entered the room. A young vascular surgeon came in to say that they had found the location of the clot. It was in my pelvic area. It was exceptionally large, and they would be admitting me to have interventional radiology remove it.

We chatted for a few minutes, and the next doctor knelt by the side of the bed. He said, "We have some bad news."

The doctor's words, delivered with a carefully constructed façade of professional neutrality, echoed in my ears.

"We found a large tumor in your bladder, presenting as cancer in your CT scan."

Without hesitation, I reached over to place my hand on his shoulder and said, "Everything will be all right."

Where did those words come from? He had a surprised look on his face. I believe God was speaking to me and through me. I remained quiet and looked around the room.

The others in the room must have expected me to break down in tears, but I did not. I had a strength I never knew I

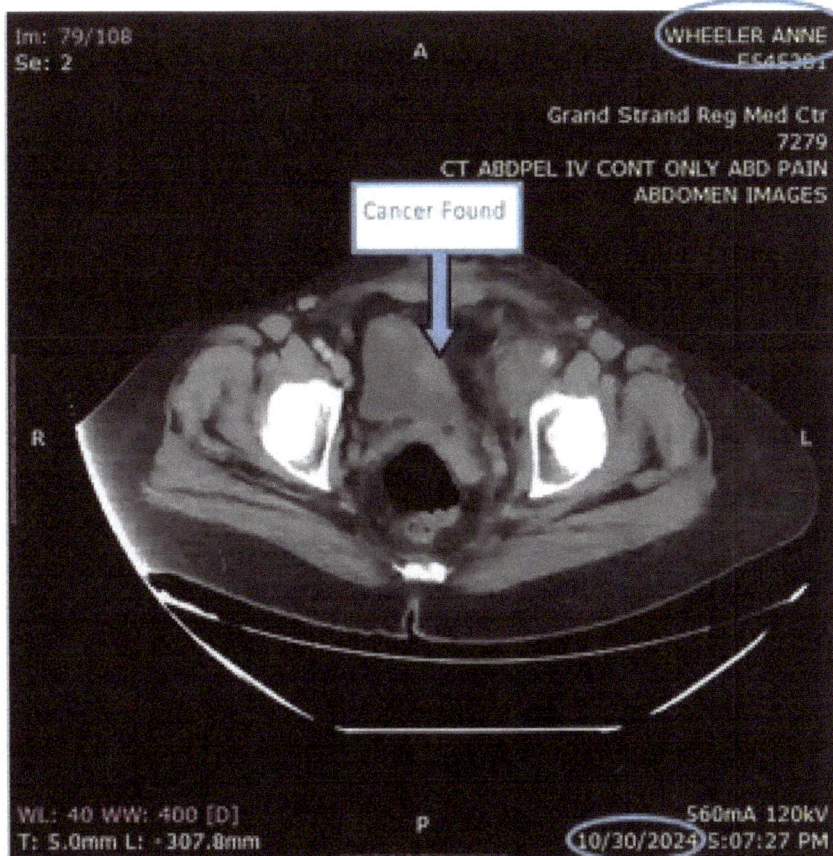

had. My faith was so strong, I just knew, inherently, God would save me from yet another cancer diagnosis. Bill, being numb at the news of yet another cancer situation, remained alert and listened to the plan to admit and remove the blood clot. Deep down, though, he panicked, he revealed later. The vascular doctor stopped by later in the evening, and we chatted about more positive things like travel and scuba diving. He also offered to show me the CT scan results, so I could see the size of the tumor. It was 5.6 cm by 2.1 cm – a good sized tumor in my small bladder.

Bill finally left to go home to take care of our two dogs. I am sure they were very confused about my absence but were happy to see Bill and get their pets and snuggles before bedtime.

The next morning, I was moved to a room in the ICU (intensive care unit). Bill and I were both exhausted from lack of sleep the night before. Once I was settled in and all the nurses had completed their duties, we both fell fast asleep for an hour or so. We were awakened by a doctor visit to prepare me for the insertion of a catheter to disperse clot-dissolving drugs.

The procedure plan was to attack the blood clot from the side of the blockage so that the next day they could suction out the clot. I was taken to the operating room and administered pain killing drugs. An incision was made behind my left knee into the main artery, and a catheter was inserted. I remained awake through all of this. If all goes well, the clot would be gone the next day, and all would be well again.

Not so fast. I still had to deal with the cancer now growing in my bladder. *Okay*, I told myself, *God has this. One problem at a time*. Each time I got overwhelmed with the issues, I asked God to give me strength. I sure needed it. The procedure went well, and I was wheeled to my room. Bill was waiting for me and gave me a big kiss. I was and am so thankful to have him by my side.

I was required to remain on my back until the next day and unable to move. It was to keep the catheter in place and distribute the clot destroying medicine and the incision to remain intact. I struggled to keep my leg immobile, especially through the night. The nurses were great and found a leg brace to assist me in keeping my leg straight and unable to bend it. It helped me rest without fear of moving while asleep. Although do you really get any rest or sleep with an automatic blood pressure cuff that goes on and off every hour and the beeps and sounds from the machines monitoring? It is not an easy task to rest or sleep in the hospital.

My faith, once my unwavering anchor, felt like a frayed rope, threatening to snap under the strain. The comforting assurances I had received from one of my pastors who visited and the strength I had derived from prayer seemed to have waned.

The whispers of doubt, once easily silenced, now roared in my ears, a relentless chorus questioning God's plan and His mercy. Why, after such a miraculous recovery would this happen again? Had I somehow failed? Had I not been faithful enough? Would God abandon me this time?

The next day it was time to remove the catheter, and the blood clot should be dissolved. It was to be an hour-long procedure. The drugs administered to numb the pain and the imaging showed that the clot had not changed; it was still the large size it was before. This told the doctors that the clot had been there for a while, and they needed to get it out quickly and safely. They injected me with contrast and did another

CT scan. This revealed that I had a different venous system that was not normal (less than 1% of the U.S. population has different venous systems).

As it turns out, this additional venous system kept blood flowing to my major organs and kept me alive even with a blood clot growing over several weeks.

I could hear the doctors discussing a plan of action. It seemed to take forever. Fear began to set in, and I asked to be told what the plan was. I assured them I would be okay if I had the information. With me, knowledge is power to overcome fear. They explained what they were going to do. I said to please be sure to give me more pain meds as what they gave me was now wearing off.

The plan was to go in through the artery behind my right knee. They would insert a disc to block this newly found venous system and a screen in the main artery to allow the blood to flow and block any clot pieces from heading north to my heart, lungs, and brain. A clot to any of my major organs would kill me. The nurse administered more pain meds, but there was not enough time to take effect before they cut behind my right knee and began to insert the necessary items.

At this point, I could feel it all and let out a whale of a groan from the pain. Tears flowed as I attempted to endure the pain and keep myself under control. I was clenching the OR (operating room) table and sheet, trying to be still and quiet. I was unable to withhold my sobbing. Eventually, the pain meds helped, but it was not soon enough.

After they inserted a tool to tear up the clot and sucked the clot pieces out, the nurse showed me the two pans of the clot pieces. It was obviously an exceptionally large clot. I was thankful for God's guidance for the doctors in resolving this exceedingly difficult procedure. What was supposed to be a one hour procedure turned into three hours but was worth the wait. I am alive and thankful to God for giving me grace through the uncertainty and pain.

Bill was waiting for me when I arrived back in my room. He had been briefed throughout the procedure by the doctor as to the progress. He was so thankful I was okay and stayed with me until late afternoon. Then he left to take care of our dogs once again.

After he left, a urology doctor came by my room to discuss the situation with my bladder cancer. He mentioned to me that I would be on blood thinners for three months and, therefore, doing any surgery to remove or biopsy the cancer would have to wait for three months. I did not say anything to him except I understood. I was not up for arguing the fact that three months is a long time for cancer to grow and get worse. When Bill returned for the evening, I explained what I was told, and we both agreed we would find a way to handle the cancer situation sooner rather than later.

Within a week, I made an appointment with my GP (General Practitioner) to discuss my situation. The procedure would be to "bridge medicate," which is to take blood thinner pills each day until two days before surgery and then change to an injection. Doing so would lessen the bleed-out risk. After the procedure, I would return to pills to finish out the three-month requirement.

My GP and I would work quickly to get a urologist to do the procedure soon. Within a couple of days, I obtained a urology doctor's appointment with a noticeably young doctor and who was new to the practice. We discussed a plan to go into my bladder to biopsy the tumor and scheduled an operating room at the hospital for a week later. Our prayers were answered. God was with us to help us get what we needed quickly.

On the morning of the "cystoscopy with biopsy," we went to the hospital and went through the normal steps for pre-op procedures. Bill went to the waiting room when I went in for the biopsy. I woke up in the post op room and noticed Bill's jacket was already there. A few minutes later, he showed up with a concerned smile on his face.

He asked if I knew what had happened and if the doctor had said anything to me. I was still coming out of my drug-induced sleep but was curious what had happened. As it turned out, the doctor went in to do the biopsy and found nothing: no tumor, no cancer, no remnants of anything. It was a healthy bladder. In the waiting room, Bill had questioned the doctor to see if she reviewed the CT scan prior to the surgery, and she said, "Yes," adding that the senior partners also reviewed it with her. The doctor was so shocked that the tumor had disappeared ("Relationship").

To be sure it was not elsewhere, the doctor performed a pelvic exam to see if the cancer was there. It was not. While it was great news, Bill and I could not wrap our heads around it. It was a true miracle – spontaneous remission.

Praise be to God!

We went to eat after I was checked out of the hospital and just sat there in happy shock. We questioned the CT scan at the hospital. Was it someone else that day that had my cancer? The CT showed the clot and the cancer, so what were the chances? Bill was told in the waiting room by my urologist that they had the same questions. During the cystoscopy procedure, the doctor called in the radiologist who did the CT scan that day, and they verified it was me.

We were just in shock and disbelief but were overwhelmed with thankfulness and happiness. God had His hand in this, and my faith in Him became even stronger. While my husband, Bill, believes in God, he struggled about the outcome. I jokingly call him my *doubting Thomas*. Bill has a strong belief in scientific facts, even though he has faith in God. To double check, we both agreed to get another CT scan to verify the science. I requested a CT scan at the cancer center just to appease him, and frankly, I wanted a follow-up scan to be able to share my miracle.

A week later, I had a follow-up with my urologist to review what she saw during the cystoscopy. They tested my urine to see if there was any blood or other matter. The doctor entered the room, and the first words out of her mouth were, "You must be my first anomaly."

I chuckled and asked questions to see if there was any scientific reason that a tumor would show up and then disappear. The doctor could not produce anything to explain it. The doctor told me the CT scan images were reviewed with the senior partners before the cystoscopy; the doctor went in and found nothing. There was no residual of a tumor or anything else. There were no remnants of blood clot or cyst either. My bladder looked healthy. The doctor told me a pelvic exam was performed, and all was good there too. I told the doctor that God had healed me again. This was truly miraculous.

Then came the day that defied all medical logic, a day that will be forever etched into my memory. The blood tests, urine tests, the attempted biopsy, and the CT scan—all showed no trace of cancer. Vanished. Gone. The doctors were baffled. My heart knew the truth.

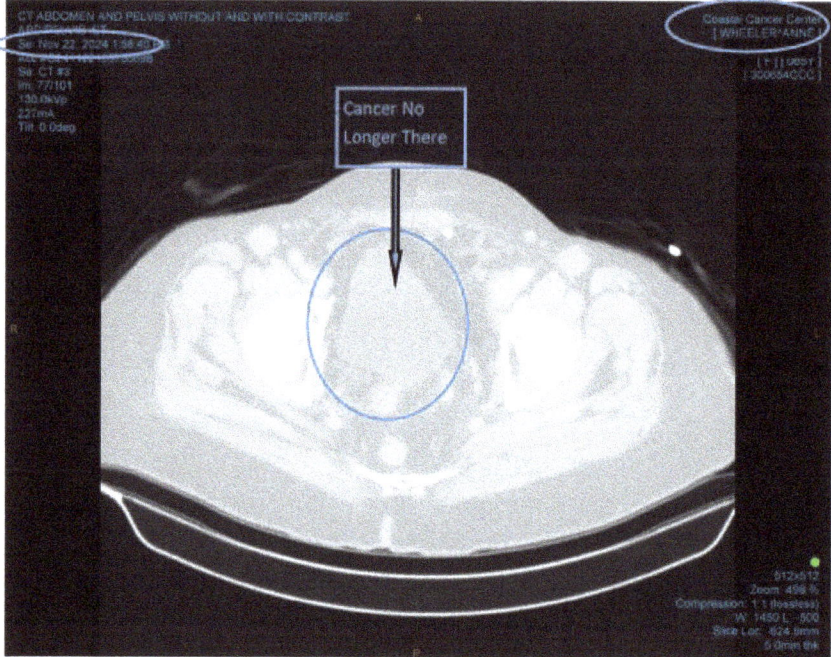

This was not a medical marvel, but a divine miracle. It was an answer to my prayers, a testament to the enduring power of faith, even amid the depths of doubt.

It was about navigating life's storms with grace, even amid the doubt. It was about acknowledging the pain, the anger, the uncertainty without allowing it to consume me entirely. It was about surrendering my will to God, allowing myself to be vulnerable, allowing myself to be broken and remade.

So do not fear, for I am with you; do not be dismayed,
for I am your God. I will strengthen you and help you;
I will uphold you with my righteous right hand.
—Isaiah 41:10 (NIV)

CHAPTER 5

My Altered Perspective on Life

*So we have come to know and to believe the love
that God has for us. God is love, and whoever abides in love
abides in God, and God abides in him.*
—1 John 4:16 (ESV)

My spiritual practices evolved. I learned to appreciate the small miracles of each day: the beauty of the sunrise, the warmth of the sun on my skin, and the laughter of my friends. These simple joys provided a grounding presence, a reminder that life, despite its challenges, was still beautiful, still precious. It was not a complete absence of fear; the specter of recurrence still haunted me. But the experience taught me the profound power of vulnerability, the beauty of letting go, the transformative power of trust in a God Who works in mysterious ways.

My faith, tested and refined in the crucible of suffering, emerged stronger, deeper, more profoundly personal than ever before. The journey had been arduous, filled with pain, doubt, and uncertainty. But amid the darkness, I had found a light, a guiding star that would illuminate my path forward.

This was not the end of my story, but a new beginning – a fresh chapter filled with hope, gratitude, and an unwavering faith in the power of divine intervention. The unexpected recurrence, and its even more unexpected resolution, had forever altered my perspective on life, death, and the miraculous power of faith. It had taught me the importance of perseverance, the beauty of vulnerability, and the unending love of a God who never truly abandons His children.

So we fix our eyes not on what is seen,
but on what is unseen, since what is seen is temporary,
but what is unseen is eternal.
—2 Corinthians 4:18 (NIV)

CHAPTER 6

Honesty in Faith

And he said to them, "Why are you troubled,
and why do doubts arise in your hearts?
—Luke 24:38 (ESV)

My journey with cancer was not a spotless march toward miraculous healing. It was messy, chaotic, and riddled with moments of profound doubt, fear, and even anger. There were times when my faith felt like a fragile thread, stretched thin against the relentless pressure of illness and uncertainty. I want to be clear: this is not a story of unwavering, perfect faith. It is a story of a very imperfect person finding strength in an unwavering God, despite the imperfections within.

It is crucial to acknowledge that faith is not a shield against suffering; it is not a magic formula that erases pain or guarantees a miraculous outcome. It is a relationship, a journey of trust and surrender, even when the path is unclear and the destination uncertain. My experience taught me that faith thrives in vulnerability, not in flawless performance. The cracks in my faith, the moments of doubt and despair, became the very spaces where God's grace could flow in and heal the deepest wounds.

My imperfections were not erased; they were embraced. I learned that God's love does not depend on my ability to maintain a constant state of spiritual perfection. It is a love that embraces my flaws, my fears, my doubts – all the messy, human elements that make me who I am. In fact, it was through the acknowledgment of my imperfections, through my honest struggles with faith, that I experienced a deeper connection with God. I began to see my vulnerabilities, not as weaknesses, but as opportunities for grace.

The struggle with doubt is not a sign of weak faith; it is a sign of a living faith grappling with the complexities of life. Many times, I felt like a child clinging to my father's hand during a thunderstorm. Fearful questioning, yet desperately needing that connection, that assurance that everything would be okay. It was not always easy. There were screams into the pillow, silent tears shed in the quiet of the night, moments where I questioned everything. But in those moments of vulnerability, I found a deeper intimacy with God. The honest confession of my doubts became a powerful act of faith.

My faith journey is not linear; it is a winding road with twists, turns, and unexpected detours. There were times when I felt overwhelmingly close to God, experiencing moments of profound peace and joy. And then there were those long, dark nights filled with doubt and despair, where the presence of God felt distant, almost imperceptible. But even in the darkness, even in the depths of my suffering, I clung to the belief that God was with me. That faith, that unwavering belief, became my lifeline, sustaining me through the storm.

Sharing this experience, this imperfect journey of faith, has been a significant part of my healing process. For so long,

I felt ashamed of my doubts, my struggles, and my past mistakes. I thought my faith had to be perfect, that I had to have all the answers. I believed that only those with unshakeable faith could experience miraculous healing. But the truth is the most profound experiences of faith often emerge from the midst of our struggles, from our honest wrestling with doubt and uncertainty.

The act of sharing my story, my imperfections and all, became a powerful tool in my healing. It allowed me to connect with others who shared similar experiences, fostering a sense of community and understanding. By acknowledging my vulnerability, I created space for others to share their own vulnerabilities without fear of judgment. We are not alone in our struggles; our shared experiences can become powerful sources of strength, hope, and healing.

The lessons I learned from embracing imperfection extended far beyond my faith. It taught me the importance of authenticity, of allowing myself to be fully seen, flaws and all. It liberated me from the burden of having to project an image of perfection. This transformation allowed me to build more genuine and meaningful relationships, both with God and with the people around me.

In my moments of weakness, I learned to lean on others for support. I discovered the incredible power of community, the strength found in shared vulnerability, and the comfort in knowing that we are not alone in our struggles. The support I received from my husband, family, friends, and church community was immeasurable. Their prayers, their unwavering support helped me navigate the darkest of times. This experience taught me the importance of reaching out for help, to lean into the love and support offered by those around me.

This journey also reinforced my belief in the power of forgiveness. Forgiveness is not just for others; it is for us as well. During my cancer journey, I had moments of anger, resentment, even bitterness. But holding onto these negative emotions only perpetuated my suffering. Learning to forgive myself for my imperfections and for my moments of doubt became a crucial step toward healing. Forgiving myself allowed me to let go of the heavy burden of guilt and shame, creating space for peace and healing to enter.

My healing, both physical and spiritual, was a slow, gradual process. It was not a sudden, dramatic transformation; rather, it was a series of small steps, moments of grace, and instances of renewed hope. Practicing gratitude helped shift my focus from my suffering to the abundance of good in my life. It grounded me in the present moment, preventing my mind from spiraling into anxiety and fear.

Practice of mindfulness became another vital tool in my healing process. Mindfulness helped me to be present in each moment and to fully experience the joy and the pain without judgment. It taught me to accept my experiences, both positive and negative, without trying to change or control them. This acceptance became a powerful source of strength, allowing me to navigate the uncertainties of my illness with greater peace and equanimity.

Through this arduous journey, I have discovered a renewed purpose in life. The cancer, the struggles, the doubts – they all served to refine my faith and to deepen my understanding of God's love and grace. I have come to cherish the small moments, to appreciate the simple joys of life, and to recognize the profound beauty in imperfection. I have found a new appreciation for the gift of life, an understanding of the preciousness of each day.

The journey continues, and I know that there will be future challenges. But armed with my faith, my resilience, and the lessons learned from embracing imperfection, I face the future with hope and optimism. My story is not a testament to flawless piety, but a testament to the enduring power of faith, even amid the imperfections of life. It is a story of hope, resilience, and the transformative power of grace. It is a story of healing, both physical and spiritual, a journey that continues to unfold, a testament to the unwavering love and grace of a God Who embraces our imperfections and walks alongside us every step of the way.

But he said to me, "My grace is sufficient for you, for my power is made perfect in weakness." Therefore I will boast all the more gladly about my weaknesses, so that Christ's power may rest on me.
—2 Corinthians 12:9 (NIV)

CHAPTER 7

Sharing Your Story

Do not neglect to do good and to share what you have,
for such sacrifices are pleasing to God.
—Hebrews 13:16 (ESV)

For a long time, I wrestled with the idea of sharing my story. The vulnerability felt immense. To expose the raw, un-filtered details of my cancer journey, the fear, the doubt, the moments where my faith felt like a flickering candle in a hur-ricane – it felt terrifying. I was used to presenting a polished version of myself: the strong, resilient survivor. But that was not the whole truth. The truth was messy, chaotic, and full of imperfections. And yet, I knew, deep down, that the very imperfections were part of the miracle.

My initial hesitation stemmed from a fear of judgment.

- Would people question my faith if I admitted to the moments of doubt?
- Would they see my vulnerability as a weakness?
- Would my story resonate if it were not a pristine nar-rative of unwavering belief and instantaneous healing?

These questions haunted me, whispering doubts that threatened to silence my voice. But then I remembered the countless others who had walked similar paths, grappling with their own illnesses, their own anxieties, their own questions of faith. I remembered the comfort I had found in the stories of others, their honesty and vulnerability offering a lifeline during my darkest hours. That is when I realized that my story, with all its imperfections, might be the very thing someone else desperately needed to hear.

Sharing my story was not about boasting about divine intervention; it was about offering a hand to those walking through the valley of the shadow of death. It was about creating a space where others could feel seen, understood, and validated in their own struggles. It was about demonstrating that faith is not about flawless piety or unwavering certainty; it is about a relationship, a journey filled with peaks and valleys, moments of unwavering faith, and moments of crippling doubt. It is a journey that acknowledges the messiness of life and the power of grace to carry us through.

The power of vulnerability lies in its authenticity. When we share our true stories, warts, and all, we create a space for connection and empathy. It is in the cracks, the imperfections, and the moments of doubt that we find the deepest resonance with others. Sharing my experience was not about presenting a perfect picture of faith; it was about offering a realistic glimpse into the heart of a struggle. It was about acknowledging that it is okay to not have all the answers, to question, to doubt, to feel overwhelmed. In fact, it is in these moments of vulnerability that faith often shines the brightest ("Share Your Story").

This journey has taught me that faith is not a shield against suffering but a companion through it. It is not about avoiding pain or hardship but finding strength and meaning amid them. My experience was not a linear progression of healing and faith. There were times when the pain was overwhelming, when fear consumed me, when my faith wavered. These were not failures of faith; they were integral parts of the journey. Sharing these moments, the moments of doubt and despair, allow others to understand that they are not alone in their struggles. Their doubts, their fears, their questions are valid and understandable.

One of the most powerful aspects of sharing my story has been the unexpected connections it has fostered. I have received countless messages from people who have shared their own struggles, their own stories of faith and healing, and their own moments of doubt. These connections have been profoundly healing, both for me and for them. The act of sharing, of being vulnerable, has created a sense of community, a network of support and understanding, where people feel safe to share their most intimate and painful experiences.

Think of the stories in the Bible–are they filled with only flawless, saintly characters? No. We see the struggles of Abraham, the doubts of Moses, and the betrayals of Peter. These stories resonate with us, not because they portray perfect people, but because they portray real people wrestling with real faith. These were individuals who, like me, experienced moments of doubt, despair, and uncertainty, yet they found strength and redemption through their relationship with God. Their stories, filled with imperfections, inspire hope because they show that faith is not about perfection; it is about perseverance, about trust even amid storms.

The support I received was overwhelming. People shared their stories of struggle and resilience. Doctors, friends, even strangers offered words of encouragement, prayers, and practical help. It was collective support, fueled by shared vulnerability, which provided the strength to navigate the uncertainty of a second cancer diagnosis. It was a powerful reminder that we are not meant to walk this journey alone. The sharing of experiences, the mutual vulnerability, created an incredible sense of community and hope ("Relationship").

The unexpected disappearance–the second miracle–further solidified the importance of vulnerability. My story, far from being a polished narrative of unwavering faith, was a testament to the power of God's grace amid imperfection. It is not about a life free from hardship, but about a relationship that sustains us through them. The journey is still unfolding; I remain acutely aware that future challenges might lie ahead. But I'll face them with a deepened sense of faith, knowing that my imperfections do not disqualify me from God's love and grace. Instead, they are the very things that make my story and the stories of others so powerfully relatable and hopeful.

My vulnerability became a bridge to connect with others. It became a way to offer comfort and hope, not by presenting a flawless image, but by showing the raw, honest reality of my journey. I share my story not as a testimony to perfect faith, but as an invitation to engage in the messy, beautiful, imperfect journey of faith with all its struggles, doubts, and triumphs. It is a journey of shared humanity, a testament to the power of vulnerability, and an affirmation of the unwavering love of God. It is a story of ongoing healing, both physical and spiritual, a journey I am committed to sharing because it is in the sharing that the true power of faith is revealed.

My hope is that by sharing the full spectrum of my experience, the moments of fear and doubt, alongside the moments of faith and hope, I can provide a beacon of encouragement for others. It is not about a perfect faith but a genuine faith;

it is not about a perfect life but a life lived in relationship with a God who embraces us in our imperfections.

This is not just my story; it is a reflection of the shared human experience, a journey of vulnerability, faith, and the unwavering power of grace. It is an invitation to embrace your own vulnerability and share your story, knowing that in doing so, you, too, can offer comfort, hope, and inspiration to others walking a similar path. The beauty of shared experiences lies in its power to connect, heal, and inspire, reminding us that we are never truly alone in our struggles. The power of vulnerability lies not in its weakness but in its strength, its honesty, and its profound capacity to build bridges of connection and hope. My journey continues, and I am profoundly grateful for the opportunity to share it, imperfections and all. For it is in our imperfections that the true strength of our faith is revealed ("Share Your Story").

But someone will say, "You have faith; I have deeds."
Show me your faith without deeds, and
I will show you my faith by my deeds.
—James 2:18 (NIV)

CHAPTER 8
Overcoming Resentment and Anger

Fear not, for I am with you; be not dismayed, for I am your God; I will strengthen you, I will help you, I will uphold you with my righteous right hand.
—Isaiah 41:10 (ESV)

The miracle of my healing was not just about the disappearance of cancer cells; it was about the transformation that occurred within my heart and soul, the journey from bitterness and resentment to forgiveness and peace. This inner healing allowed me to approach life with renewed purpose, to appreciate the preciousness of each day, and to share my story of hope and healing with others. My journey was a testament to the power of faith, not perfect faith, but a real faith, a faith that allowed me to find grace, strength, and healing amid the storms of adversity. And in sharing this journey, my hope is that you, too, might find your path to forgiveness and discover the profound peace that comes with letting go. The journey to healing, both physical and spiritual, is a testament to the power of faith, perseverance, and the unwavering support of loved ones and faith.

The unexpected recurrence of cancer in 2024 and its equally inexplicable disappearance further deepened my understanding of the mystery and grace that underpins life. The medical community remains baffled, unable to offer a scientific explanation for this anomaly. But for me, it serves as a testament to the power of faith and the inexplicable workings of God. It is a reminder that life is full of surprises, that hope can emerge even in the darkest of hours, and that faith can provide comfort and strength that transcends the limitations of human understanding. This experience reaffirmed the importance of trust, not just in medical science, but in the unwavering presence of God in my life, an unseen force that guided and sustained me through the chaos. The experience reinforced the idea that my recovery was not just a medical phenomenon, but a miraculous event guided by divine intervention ("Coping").

My journey has not ended. It is an ongoing process, a constant unfolding of lessons learned, perspectives gained, and faith deepened. Each day presents new challenges and new opportunities for growth. But through it all, I carry with me the lessons learned, the unwavering faith that has sustained me, and the deep sense of gratitude for the life I have been given, a life infused with a newfound appreciation for the simple yet profound blessings that surround us.

My hope is that

- my story will resonate with others facing similar challenges, offering messages of hope, resilience, and the enduring power of faith in the face of adversity.
- others will discover their own path to healing and wholeness, finding strength in their imperfections,

and discovering the boundless love and unwavering support that surrounds them.

- they will find their own path to faith, a faith that transcends doubt and strengthens the human spirit in its darkest hours.

It is faith that empowers us to find peace, purpose, and healing. And it is a faith that, for me, continues to blossom with each passing day.

> *When the righteous thrive, the people rejoice;*
> *when the wicked rule, the people groan.*
> *—Proverbs 29:2 (NIV)*

CHAPTER 9
The Role of Belief

Because, if you confess with your mouth that Jesus is Lord and believe in your heart that God raised him from the dead, you will be saved. For with the heart one believes and is justified, and with the mouth one confesses and is saved.
—Romans 10:9-10 (ESV)

For all its advancements, modern science often struggles to fully comprehend the intricate dance between the mind and body. We know that stress, anxiety, and negative emotions can weaken our immune systems, making us more vulnerable to illness. Conversely, positive emotions, a sense of purpose, and strong social connections can bolster our resilience and promote healing. This is not merely a matter of *thinking positively*; it is about fostering a deep internal shift in perspective, a shift that fundamentally alters our physiological responses.

Countless studies have demonstrated the link between mental states and physical health outcomes. The placebo effect, for instance, highlights the power of belief itself to influence our physical experience. Patients given a sugar pill, believing it to be a potent medication, often experience real, measurable improvements in their symptoms. This is not about deception; it is about the remarkable ability of the mind to impact the body.

My own experience underscored this connection. During my first battle with cancer, the constant fear and anxiety undoubtedly took a toll. The fatigue, the lack of sleep, and the exhaustion, were amplified by the constant worry. However, as my faith deepened, as I surrendered my anxieties to God, I found a surprising strength. Prayer was not just a ritual; it was a conscious act of releasing my fears and placing my trust in God. This act, in turn, had a tangible effect on my physical well-being. I found myself sleeping better and possessing a renewed sense of energy.

Prayer has been the subject of numerous scientific studies. While the mechanisms are not fully understood, research suggests that prayer can have measurable benefits for both physical and mental health. Some studies have shown a correlation between prayer and improved cardiovascular health, while others have demonstrated its effectiveness in reducing anxiety and depression ("Mindfulness Meditation").

During my second diagnosis, the reappearance of cancer after such a miraculous removal of all the cancer in the initial biopsy, I did not grapple with doubt. I felt that everything would be okay. God had given me His grace in my first cancer diagnosis, which was an early diagnosis, was that I didn't require radiation or chemotherapy. I was spared for a reason. What that reason was, I knew in time. I would discover what God's plan was for me. It was not a simple, unwavering belief, but a more mature and resilient faith with an ounce of uncertainty. The power of prayer deepened during this period, not to magically erase the cancer, but to find solace, strength, and a sense of connection with God amid uncertainty. It was a form of surrender, acceptance, and an unwavering belief in God's unwavering love ("Relationship").

The subsequent disappearance of the second cancer, inexplicable to my doctors, reinforced the power of this mind-body-God connection. It was not just faith that healed me; it was the interplay between faith and my conscious effort to nurture my mental and spiritual well-being. It was not about choosing between faith and science; it was about integrating them. After all, God created science and us in His image with the abilities to create the tools and treatment, but my faith and spiritual practices provided the mental and emotional resilience needed to navigate the storm. My unwavering belief in God's plan, coupled with the support of my loving husband and my faith community, profoundly impacted my healing journey. These aspects, while intangible, were integral to the overall outcome.

This understanding of the mind-body connection is not merely anecdotal; it is supported by a growing body of scientific evidence. The burgeoning field of psychoneuroimmunology explores the intricate interplay between the brain, the nervous system, and the immune system. It demonstrates that psychological factors, such as stress and anxiety, can have a significant impact on our immune responses. This knowledge has profound implications for cancer patients, highlighting the importance of managing stress, nurturing positive emotions, and finding solace in spiritual practices that enhance mental and emotional well-being ("Psychoneuroimmunology").

In my own case, it was the unwavering belief in God, the strength found in prayer and meditation, and the overwhelming support of my faith community that gave me the strength to fight the illness, not just physically, but mentally and spiritually. This holistic approach is what I believe significantly contributed to my healing ("Supporting").

My experience is not intended to diminish the importance of conventional medical care. Throughout my journey, I worked closely with a dedicated team of doctors and medical professionals. Their expertise and skills were essential in my care and recovery. Faith and medical care are not mutually exclusive; they are complementary. Faith provided the emotional and spiritual strength to endure the challenges of medical care, while medical care provided the necessary interventions to address the physical aspects of my illness. Together, they were a powerful force in my healing.

The road to healing is not always linear. There will be setbacks, moments of doubt, and times when faith feels like a distant whisper. But even in those moments, it is crucial to cultivate hope and perseverance. These qualities, along with proactive lifestyle choices that support physical and mental health, are essential elements in the healing process. It is a journey that requires both inner and outer work, a delicate balance of medical intervention and conscious attention to the mind-body connection. It is a testament to the intricate and often unseen forces that shape our experiences and the profound impact that faith, hope, and an unwavering belief in a higher power can have on our physical well-being. My journey is a testament to the incredible capacity of the human spirit, the strength found in faith, and the undeniable reality of the mind-body-God connection ("Mindfulness Meditation").

For it is with your heart that you believe and are justified, and it is with your mouth that you profess your faith and are saved.
—Romans 10:10 (NIV)

CHAPTER 10

Scientific Perspectives

*Therefore confess your sins to each other and pray
for each other so that you may be healed. The prayer of
a righteous person is powerful and effective.*
—James 5:16 (NIV)

My journey through cancer, twice over, was a profound exploration of the intricate dance between faith, science, and the remarkable capacity of the human mind and body to heal. While modern medicine played a role, I passionately believe that the power of prayer significantly contributed to my recovery. This is not about dismissing the importance of medical intervention; it is about acknowledging a holistic approach to healing, one that integrates the spiritual and the scientific.

The scientific community, once hesitant to explore the connection between spirituality and health, is now increasingly acknowledging the potential benefits of prayer and meditation. Numerous studies have investigated the physiological effects of these practices, revealing fascinating insights into their impact on stress reduction, immune function, and overall well-being. For instance, research has shown that regular meditation can lower cortisol levels–the stress hormone–which is known to suppress the immune system. Chronic stress weakens the body's defenses, making it more vulnerable to illness. By reducing stress, meditation can indirectly bolster the immune system, potentially aiding in the body's natural healing processes. This is not to say meditation cures cancer; rather, it contributes to a healthier environment within the body, allowing it to function optimally during treatment and recovery.

For many, prayer serves as a powerful tool for coping with stress and anxiety. In my case, my faith that Jesus healed many who believed in Him when He walked the earth became my focus. Jesus still heals His believers to this day. Many of His miracles have been shared throughout time and many more to this day. He healed me completely without any further care needed. That had such an impact on me, so I felt compelled to author this book to bring hope to those dealing with cancer or other major illnesses. Believe in Jesus and ask for His healing while collaborating with the doctors and nurses to assist you. God has given them the gift to help you on your journey.

The impact of prayer is more challenging to quantify scientifically. While measuring the direct physiological effects of prayer is complex, numerous studies have examined its correlation with improved mental and emotional well-being. For some people, the act of surrendering worries and concerns to a higher power can provide a sense of peace and control in the face of uncertainty, reducing feelings of helplessness and fear. This sense of peace, in turn, can have a positive cascading effect on the body's physiological processes, potentially influencing hormone levels, blood pressure, and sleep patterns – all factors crucial for healing.

One fascinating area of research explores the placebo effect in conjunction with prayer and meditation. The placebo effect, while often dismissed as a mere psychological phe-nomenon, demonstrates the remarkable power of belief in shaping physical outcomes.

Studies have shown that patients who believe they are receiving effective treatment often experience improved symptoms, even if the treatment itself is inert. Prayer and meditation can enhance the placebo effect by fostering a positive mindset and promoting a sense of hope and expec-tation for healing. The belief in a higher power, coupled with the practice of prayer and meditation, may amplify this effect, contributing to a more potent healing response.

Consider the concept of intentionality in prayer. Many be-lieve that focused prayer with specific intentions for healing can direct positive energy toward the body and mind. While this remains an area of ongoing research, the very act of focusing one's attention on healing can be empowering and potentially beneficial. This is aligned with concepts of mind-body medicine, which emphasizes the intricate connection between mental and physical states. Intentional prayer, combined with visual-ization techniques, can create a powerful synergy, amplifying the potential for healing.

My personal experience deeply reinforces the findings of these studies. During my first cancer battle, daily prayer became a lifeline. It was not a ritualistic recitation; it was a conversation with God, a pouring out of my fears, hopes, and anxieties. It was a space where I could surrender my burdens and find solace in unwavering faith ("Relationship").

Simultaneously, I incorporated meditation, finding a quiet sanctuary amid the chaos of medical care. Meditation provided a sense of calm and focus, helping me navigate the emotional rollercoaster of my illness. The combined power of prayer and meditation created a sanctuary within the storm, grounding me in faith and empowering me to face my challenges with courage and resilience.

The second time I faced a cancer diagnosis the fear was not as intense as my faith, strengthened by previous experience, remained my anchor. Prayer and some meditation, which had become habits, became even more crucial. They were not merely coping mechanisms; they were integral to my healing process. I actively sought to create a positive internal environment, conducive to healing by aligning my thoughts, emotions, and actions with my faith and my hope.

It is important to note that the scientific understanding of the interplay between faith, prayer, meditation, and physical healing is still evolving. More research is undoubtedly needed to fully elucidate the mechanisms through which these practices exert their influence. However, the existing evidence suggests a strong correlation between spiritual practices and improved health outcomes. The accumulating research demonstrates that prayer and meditation are not simply passive activities; they are active interventions that can positively impact the mind and body.

Many studies have explored the effects of intercessory prayer – prayer offered on behalf of someone else. While some studies have shown positive results, others have yielded inconclusive or negative findings. The complexities of measuring the impact of intercessory prayer are significant, including the challenges in standardizing prayer practices and defining measurable outcomes. Nevertheless, the very act of receiving prayers from loved ones can provide emotional comfort and support and strengthen the patient's sense of hope and contribute in a positive healing environment.

The experience of receiving intercessory prayer can be a powerful source of emotional strength. Knowing that others are praying for your well-being can create a sense of connection and shared purpose, lessening feelings of isolation and fostering a sense of community. This emotional support can contribute to a more positive healing environment. Even if the physiological effects of intercessory prayer are debated, the emotional benefits are undeniable. Furthermore, the incorporation of prayer and meditation into a holistic healing approach does not negate the importance of conventional medical treatment. Instead, it serves as a complementary therapy, supporting and enhancing the effectiveness of traditional medical interventions. It is a matter of integrating diverse approaches, drawing strength from both scientific advancements and spiritual practices. The aim is not to replace medical care but to enhance it by addressing the mind-body connection in a comprehensive and synergistic way.

My journey underscores the profound interconnectedness of the physical, mental, and spiritual realms. The power of prayer and meditation, while often overlooked in conventional medical approaches, offers a potent tool for healing.

It is crucial to embrace a holistic approach, recognizing the synergistic relationship between medical science and spiritual practices. My miraculous recoveries twice over stand as a testament to this truth, a powerful reminder of the transformative power of faith and the remarkable capacity of the human spirit to heal. The scientific community is gradually acknowledging the validity of this holistic approach.

While the exact mechanisms are still under investigation, the tangible benefits are increasingly difficult to ignore. My story is not just a personal narrative; it is a plea to embrace the integrated healing that lies at the intersection of science and spirituality ("Mindfulness Meditation").

> *He said to her, "Daughter, your faith has healed you.*
> *Go in peace and be freed from your suffering."*
> *—Mark 5:34 (NIV)*

CHAPTER 11
Managing Stress and Anxiety

*Cast all your anxiety on him because
he cares for you.*
—1 Peter 5:7 (NIV)

The initial shock of my cancer diagnosis in 2022 felt like a physical blow. The word itself, *cancer*, hung in the air, heavy and suffocating. Fear, raw and visceral, clawed at my insides. Anxiety, a relentless tide, threatened to pull me under. Sleep became elusive, replaced by a constant stream of terrifying *what ifs*? The medical jargon–biopsies, staging, treatment plans – blurred into a meaningless cacophony, further intensifying my distress. My rational mind understood the need for treatment, for fighting this disease with the best medical science has to offer. Yet, the emotional turmoil was overwhelming.

Amid this storm, my faith became my anchor. It was not a sudden, dramatic conversion; it was the slow, steady unfolding of a long-held belief, now tested in the crucible of fear. Prayer, which had been a comforting routine, became a lifeline. It was not about demanding a miracle; it was about surrendering my anxieties to a power greater than myself. I poured out my fears, my doubts, my raw, unfiltered pain into those silent conversations with God. And in the stillness that followed, a sense of peace, however fragile, would begin to settle.

This was not passive acceptance of my fate. It was not about ignoring the harsh realities of my illness. Instead, faith provided a framework for navigating the uncertainty, a lens through which to view my situation with a perspective that extended beyond the immediate terror. It helped me to focus on what I *could* control: my attitude, my choices regarding treatment, and my commitment to fostering hope.

The support of my faith community proved invaluable. The shared prayers, the visits, and the simple acts of kindness created a tangible network of love and support that enveloped me, cushioning the impact of my fear. The stories shared by fellow congregants, tales of their own struggles and triumphs, reminded me that I was not alone on my journey. Their unwavering faith became a source of inspiration and a tangible example of the resilience of the human spirit.

Meditation also became a part of my coping strategy. Initially, I found it challenging to quiet my racing mind to still the constant barrage of worries. But with practice, I learned to find solace in the present moment. Focusing on my breath, on the gentle rise and fall of my chest, allowed me to detach, if only for a few precious minutes, from the anxieties that threatened to consume me. These moments of stillness became islands of calm in a sea of turbulence. During these meditative periods, I found myself opening up more deeply to a sense of peace and to a quieter, more reassuring form of faith. The quiet acceptance that meditation brought helped to calm my racing heart, providing a counterpoint to the chaos of my physical experience ("Mindfulness Meditation").

My experience was not just about prayer and meditation; it was also about cultivating gratitude. During the physical discomfort and the emotional turmoil, I actively sought out things to be thankful for – the love of my family, the kindness of friends, the simple beauty of a sunset. This practice was initially challenging, and it gradually became a powerful tool for shifting my perspective. By focusing on the positive aspects of my life, I was able to counterbalance the negativity that threatened to engulf me. It was like tilting the scales, gradually re-balancing the precarious equilibrium between hope and despair.

It is crucial to acknowledge that my faith did not magically erase my fear or anxiety. There were days, even weeks, when the darkness felt overwhelming, when doubt crept in, and when the weight of my illness threatened to crush me. My faith was not a shield against suffering; it was a companion and a source of strength that allowed me to navigate the storm and to find meaning even amid pain. It provided a framework for understanding my suffering, a way to see beyond the immediate crisis, to embrace the challenges with resilience, and to find the strength to continue fighting. It was in these moments of vulnerability that my faith was most profoundly tested, and it was in these moments that it proved most valuable.

The second cancer diagnosis in 2024 was even more surprising. There was no initial wave of panic amplified by the disbelief. The tools I had developed during my first battle with cancer – prayer, meditation, gratitude – were now more readily available, more deeply ingrained. This time my faith became my immediate refuge. The familiarity of these practices provided a sense of stability, a sense of control in an otherwise overwhelming and uncertain situation.

This time, the miraculous disappearance of my cancer was even more profound. It was not just a matter of remission; it was a complete and inexplicable disappearance. The doctors were baffled, but my faith had become so deeply rooted, so intimately connected to my being, that the miracle, while inexplicable through scientific means, felt entirely natural and expected. This experience reinforced the power of integrating faith into my healing journey.

The science of stress reduction and anxiety management offers compelling evidence to support my experience. Studies have shown a strong correlation between faith and reduced stress, improved mental well-being, and even enhanced physical health. The physiological effects of prayer and meditation, such as lower blood pressure and reduced cortisol levels, are increasingly well-documented. The release of endorphins, natural mood boosters, during prayer and meditation also plays a significant role in promoting a sense of well-being and reducing anxiety. These scientific findings, while not explaining the miraculous aspects of my own journey, do offer a tangible framework for understanding the positive impact of faith on both mental and physical health.

Furthermore, the social support provided by my faith community played a vital role in my emotional well-being. Social connections and a strong sense of community are essential for managing stress and improving resilience. The feeling of belonging and of being surrounded by love and support provided a powerful buffer against isolation and fear that often accompany serious illness. This social support provided a critical element in counteracting the potential detrimental effects of stress on my health.

In the context of my journey, faith was not simply a passive belief; it was an active engagement, a practice that shaped my response to stress and anxiety. It provided the structure and the tools to navigate difficult emotions, and it encouraged the development of resilience. It transformed fear into hope, despair into determination, and uncertainty into trust. This holistic approach, integrating faith with medical intervention, played a crucial role in my physical healing and in fostering a deep sense of peace and acceptance. It is a testament to the synergistic relationship between science and spirituality and a profound affirmation of the remarkable healing power of faith. The journey itself, though arduous, reaffirmed the significance of integrating this holistic approach into one's response to illness and into one's understanding of health and well-being.

My story is not intended to diminish the importance of medical treatment. I am deeply grateful for the expertise and care of my medical team. Rather, it is a testament to the power of integrating a holistic approach to healing, one that acknowledges and embraces the interplay between science and spirituality. It is a story about finding strength in faith, even amid the storm; a story about embracing hope, even in the face of fear; and a story about the transformative power of believing even in something larger than us.

My journey has taught me that true healing is multifaceted, encompassing the physical, the emotional, and the spiritual aspects of our being. It is a journey of embracing all facets of the self, trusting in the innate healing capabilities of the human spirit, and acknowledging the profound impact that a faith-based approach can have on the experience and out-come of a challenging journey, such as mine. It is a journey I encourage others who face similar experiences to embrace, to find their own path to healing, to integrate their own belief systems, and to strengthen their own personal relationship with a higher power whatever form that may take. This is my message, my hope, and the essence of my healing journey.

Therefore I tell you, do not worry about your life, what you will eat or drink; or about your body, what you will wear. Is not life more than food, and the body more than clothes?
—Matthew 6:25 (NIV)

CHAPTER 12

Integrating Faith and Science

*Clearly no one who relies on the law is justified
before God, because "the righteous will live by faith."*
—Galatians 3:11 (NIV)

T he second cancer diagnosis in 2024, the one that inexplicably disappeared, solidified my belief in the power of faith integrated with medical care. The doctors were perplexed, but my faith remained steadfast. It was not a rejection of scientific understanding, but rather a recognition that there are dimensions to healing that extend beyond the purely physical. The experience reinforced the idea that true healing is a holistic undertaking, encompassing body, mind, and spirit. It confirmed to me that faith is not an alternative to medical care, but a powerful complement to it, a source of strength and resilience in the face of adversity.

My story is not intended to provide a formula for miraculous healing; every journey is unique. It is not about promising a specific outcome but about sharing the transformative power of integrating faith into the healing process. It is a testament to the strength found in a deep relationship with God, and the profound impact that faith can have on one's journey toward health and well-being. It is a reminder that faith and science are not mutually exclusive; they are complementary forces that, when integrated, can empower individuals to face life's most daunting challenges with courage, hope, and unwavering resilience.

For those facing similar health crises, I encourage you to explore your own path toward integrating faith and medicine. Embrace the expertise of your medical team, while simultaneously nurturing your spiritual well-being. Find a community that supports you emotionally and spiritually. Engage in practices that bring you peace, joy, and a sense of connection to something larger than yourself. Remember that healing is a multifaceted process, and your faith can be a powerful ally in this journey. Do not shy away from your vulnerability; allow yourself to feel your emotions, both joy and pain. Allow your faith to be your anchor, your source of strength, and your guide toward healing and wholeness. The journey may be challenging, but it is also an opportunity for growth, transformation, and a deeper understanding of yourself and your relationship with the divine. Never underestimate the power of hope, prayer, and the unwavering support of loved ones and your faith community. These are invaluable elements in the journey towards healing, allowing you to face whatever challenges may come with strength, resilience, and peace.

Throughout my entire journey, I have found strength in the community. My family, friends, and faith community formed a protective circle of support, providing unwavering love, prayer, and practical assistance. They reminded me of my worth, encouraged me to keep fighting, and helped me navigate the emotional complexities of my illness. This support network was not simply a source of comfort; it was a vital component of my healing process. The human connection, the shared prayers, and the tangible expressions of love and support strengthened my spirit and nourished my soul.

The importance of this human connection cannot be overstated. It is crucial to surround yourself with a supportive community, a network of people who will uplift you, encourage you, and remind you of your strength. Whether that community is within your family, your faith community, or a support group, its presence is invaluable in the journey toward healing. Connecting with others who understand your experience can alleviate feelings of isolation and provide a sense of belonging. This shared experience, this mutual support, can create a powerful synergy that strengthens both individuals and the community. It fosters a sense of hope and shared purpose, a belief that together you can overcome any challenge.

You see that his faith and his actions were working together,
and his faith was made complete by what he did.
—James 2:22 (NIV)

CHAPTER 13
The Role of Perseverance and Hope

"Not only that, but we also rejoice in our sufferings, because we know that suffering produces perseverance; perseverance, character; and character, hope."
—Romans 5:3-4 (NIV)

My journey was not solely about the miraculous disappearances of cancerous cells. It was, and continues to be, a profound exploration of perseverance, hope, and the active role I played in my own healing. While I passionately believe in the power of divine intervention, I also recognize the importance of my own conscious efforts in supporting that intervention. It was not a passive waiting for a miracle; it was an active participation in my own recovery, a dance between faith and action.

The first diagnosis, the shock, the fear – those were overwhelming. But even amid the tempest of emotions, a tiny seed of hope took root. This hope was not a naive optimism; it was a deep-seated conviction, fueled by my faith that I would fight, that I would endure, and that I would emerge stronger on the other side. This was not simply a passive acceptance of faith, but an active engagement with my spiritual life.

Prayer became a lifeline, a constant connection to a power far greater than me. It was not just about asking for healing; it was about surrendering my anxieties, finding peace amid chaos, and strengthening my resolve to face each challenge head-on.

Exercise, even in its most modest forms, played a crucial role. Walking, gentle yoga, and even simple stretches helped to improve my circulation, increase my energy levels, and alleviate the fatigue that often accompanied my treatments. The physical activity also provided a much-needed outlet for stress and anxiety. Movement helped to clear my mind, allowing me to focus on the positive aspects of my life, even amid the ongoing challenges. It was not about rigorous workouts; it was about consistent movement, nurturing my body's ability to heal.

Sleep was often underestimated in the healing process, but it became a sacred priority. Adequate rest allowed my body to repair and rejuvenate itself. I established a regular sleep schedule, creating a calming bedtime routine to drift off peacefully. I learned the importance of a conducive sleep environment – darkness, quiet, and comfortable temperature. It was not merely about getting enough sleep; it was about cultivating a deep, restorative sleep that allowed my body to heal on a cellular level.

It is vital to emphasize that my approach is not a prescriptive formula. It is a testament to the power of individual journeys, the unique pathways that each person navigates on his/her own healing odyssey. There's no one-size-fits-all solution; what worked for me may not work for everyone.

What is essential is recognizing the interconnectedness of our being in and actively participating in our own healing process.

The role of hope is paramount. Hope is not simply a feeling; it is a powerful force that fuels perseverance and empowers us to act. It is the belief that healing is possible, the conviction that we can overcome adversity. Cultivating hope requires a conscious effort; it requires focusing on the positive aspects of our lives, celebrating small victories, and surrounding ourselves with supportive individuals who believe in our potential. It is about maintaining faith, not just in a higher power, but in oneself and one's ability to heal.

Perseverance is the steadfast commitment to the healing journey, the unwavering resolve to continue even when faced with setbacks and challenges. It is about recognizing that healing is not a linear process; it is a journey with twists, turns, and moments of doubt. It is about maintaining our commitment to our well-being, even when our energy wanes, and our hope feels fragile. It is about remembering our purpose, our reasons for fighting, and holding onto the vision of a healed and vibrant future ("Coping").

For the righteous falls seven times and rises again,
but the wicked stumble in times of calamity.
—Proverbs 24:16 (ESV)

CHAPTER 14

Sharing Your Testimony

"Come and hear, all you who fear God;
let me tell you what he has done for me."
—Psalm 66:16

My journey through cancer, a harrowing odyssey of physical and emotional turmoil, often leaves an indelible mark on the soul. For me, the experience was not just a battle against a disease; it was a profound spiritual awakening, a refining fire that forged a deeper, more intimate relationship with God. And in the crucible of that experience, a quiet conviction emerged: I needed to share my story – not just for my own healing, but to offer solace, hope, and a testament to the enduring power of faith to those navigating similar storms.

This was not a decision I reached easily. Initially, the vulnerability terrified me. Sharing my deepest fears, my moments of doubt, my raw, unfiltered emotional landscape was about wanting to expose a wound that had barely begun to heal. The fear of judgment, of being misunderstood, held me captive. Would people believe my account of miraculous intervention? Would they dismiss it as mere coincidence, a lucky break, or a statistical anomaly? These questions haunted me.

But God, in His infinite wisdom, gently nudged me forward. He whispered encouragement through the prayers of loved ones, through the shared testimonies of fellow cancer survivors, and through the quiet promptings of my own heart. The more I prayed, the more I realized that my story was not just **my story.** It was a piece of a larger narrative, a testament to God's unwavering love and grace, a beacon of hope for those lost in the darkness of despair.

The pivotal moment came during a Christian ladies LIFE luncheon meeting. I sat listening over the last few years to the stories of survival from devastating accidents and cancer, and of God's grace in helping people through their life challenges, their voices laced with fear, uncertainty, and profound sadness. Their struggles mirrored mine, and in that shared vulnerability, a powerful connection was forged. It was in that space, surrounded by others who understood the depth of pain, sadness, and God's hand in helping them, that I felt emboldened to speak ("Sharing").

I began to share fragments of my journey, hesitant at first, my voice trembling slightly. But as I spoke, a transformation occurred. The weight on my chest lifted, replaced by a sense of lightness, of freedom. And what happened next surprised me even more. Others, inspired by my vulnerability, began to share their own stories, their own struggles, their own encounters with God's grace. The room, once filled with a palpable sense of sadness, was transformed into a space of hope, healing, and shared faith.

This experience was a turning point. Then I understood the profound power of sharing our testimonies. Our stories, raw and unfiltered, have the power to connect us, to comfort us, to remind us that we are not alone in our struggles. They offer a lifeline of hope, a testament to the resilience of the human spirit, and a powerful reminder of God's unwavering love.

Finding your voice, however, is not always easy. For some, it might feel like a mountain to climb, a daunting task that requires immense courage and vulnerability. For others, the fear of judgment or misunderstanding might feel insurmountable. But I want to assure you that the journey of sharing your story is worthwhile. It is a testament to your strength, a declaration of your faith, and a profound act of service to others ("Sharing").

Here are some practical steps to help you find your voice:

Start small: You do not have to share your entire life story at once. Begin by sharing small snippets of your journey with trusted friends and family. Their support and encouragement can provide the foundation you need to build your confidence.

Write it down: Sometimes, putting your thoughts and feelings on paper can be easier than speaking to them aloud. Journaling can be a powerful tool for processing emotions, clarifying thoughts, and discovering the narrative thread of your story.

Join a support group: Connecting with others, who share similar experiences, can provide a safe and supportive environment for sharing your story. Listening to others' stories can also help you find your own voice and feel less alone.

Practice: Like any skill, sharing your testimony requires practice. Start by telling your story to a small group of people, then gradually expand your audience as your confidence grows.

Embrace imperfection: Your story does not have to be perfect. It is okay to be vulnerable, to admit your mistakes, and to acknowledge your doubts. Authenticity is key. People connect with honesty and vulnerability more than polished perfection.

Pray for guidance: Seek God's guidance and wisdom as you navigate this journey. Ask Him to help you find the right words to share your story with compassion and empathy and to use your story to touch the lives of others ("Mindfulness Meditation").

·· •●• ··

Beyond personal healing, sharing your testimony offers a powerful means to inspire others. Your experience, no matter how challenging, can become a source of strength and hope for those facing similar difficulties. By sharing your journey of faith and healing, you are not merely recounting your experiences; you are extending a hand of compassion, offering encouragement, and sharing a message of hope that can transform lives.

Consider the impact of your story: For someone battling cancer, your words might offer a lifeline of hope, a testament to the possibility of healing, and a reassurance that they are not alone. For those struggling with their faith, your journey could illuminate the transformative power of prayer, the unwavering presence of God even in the darkest of times. For those wrestling with doubt, your story could offer a glimpse of the resilience of the human spirit, the strength that emerges when we surrender to God's plan.

Remember, your story is unique, valuable, and powerful. It is a gift you can share with the world, a message of hope that can inspire and transform lives. Do not underestimate the impact of your voice, the healing power of your testimony and the profound difference you can make by simply sharing your truth.

The act of sharing is not solely about speaking to others; it is also about processing your own experience, confronting lingering fears, and consolidating your own faith. The more you articulate your journey, the more clarity you gain, and the stronger your faith becomes. This process is not just about inspiring others; it is a crucial part of your own continuous healing.

Think about the ways you can share your story. Perhaps you could write a blog post, create a video testimonial, speak at a support group, or simply share your story with friends and family. There are countless avenues to share your experience; find what resonates most with you and your personality. Remember, even a simple conversation can have a profound impact.

Beyond sharing your personal testimony, consider other ways to inspire others. Volunteer at a local hospital, offer support to a friend or family member going through a difficult time, or simply offer a kind word or gesture to someone in need. These acts of service not only benefit others, but they also strengthen your own faith and deepen your sense of purpose. Personally, I found my volunteer work with my therapy dog, Bella, at my own cancer center, an experience that gives me strength while sharing love and hope through Bella to those being infused. The patients' appreciation for what I do there reminds me that my journey has a purpose beyond personal healing – it is a ministry of hope.

Finding your voice is a journey, a path of self-discovery and spiritual growth. It is a path that requires courage, vulnerability, and faith. But trust me, the rewards are immeasurable.

Your story has the power to inspire, heal, and transform not only your own life, but the lives of countless others. Embrace your story, share your truth, and let your voice become a beacon of hope in a world that desperately needs it. The world needs your story. God has a plan for your voice, and it is a powerful one. So, find it, nurture it, and share it with the world ("Sharing").

Because of the service by which you have proved yourselves, others will praise God for the obedience that accompanies your confession of the gospel of Christ, and for your generosity in sharing with them and with everyone else.
—2 Corinthians 9:13 (NIV)

CHAPTER 15

Connecting with Others

The LORD himself goes before you and will be with you;
he will never leave you nor forsake you. Do not be afraid;
do not be discouraged"
—Deuteronomy 31:8 (NIV)

Finally, leaving a legacy of faith is not simply about what we do but also about what we share. Sharing our stories, both triumphs and challenges, allows us to connect with others on a deeper level, fostering a sense of community and mutual support. By sharing our experiences of faith, we provide inspiration and hope to others who may be struggling.

We create a space for vulnerability, understanding, and shared growth. By being open and honest about our journey, we inspire others to embrace their own unique paths and to find strength in their faith. This openness and vulnerability create a powerful ripple effect, inspiring others to live their own purposeful lives, guided by their faith.

The act of sharing, of connecting with others on a spiritual level, is a vital component of leaving a legacy of faith ("Sharing").

Carry each other's burdens, and in this way
you will fulfill the law of Christ.
—Galatians 6:2 (NIV)

Inspiring Others

*"Therefore encourage one another and build
each other up, just as in fact you are doing."*
—1 Thessalonians 5:11(NIV)

If you believe that God has never been a part of your life and that you do not know where to start, think back. God is always with you. Did you ever arrive in a situation where you thought *WHEW! I just missed getting killed or injured* or you heard a voice in your head that told you to do something to avoid a bad situation? Some people call this a sixth sense, but it is the Holy Spirit or one of God's angels watching over you and guiding you.

During a time when I was not as close to God as I am now, I experienced a mind-blowing experience. One of my friends and neighbors was killed in a head on car crash. My heart hurt for his loss and for his wife and children. He had three young children under the age of five with one on the way. I struggled for several days, unable to keep tears away. I was unable to sleep well. One night while I was asleep, I was awakened by a bright light in the shape of a figure. I sat up in bed, and as the figure spoke to me with a British female voice, I heard, "You can stop crying now. He is in a great place." As the bright light disappeared, I laid my head back down and fell fast asleep. I never forgot that time that God sent an angel to help me through my sadness. I believe the light before me was my deceased Aunt Anne, who hailed from the UK.

I am sure you have experienced little miracles in your life that God shows His love for you. Think of those little miracles and get started asking God to help you. Talk to Him as if He were your friend because He is.

He is always there to help you. You just need to ask.

"The LORD himself goes before you and will be with you;
he will never leave you nor forsake you.
Do not be afraid; do not be discouraged."
—Deuteronomy 31:8 (NIV)

Acknowledgments

This book would not have been possible without the unwavering support and love of my incredible husband, family, and friends. Their prayers, encouragement, and unwavering belief in me sustained me through the darkest hours.

- My deepest gratitude goes to my husband, Bill, for his tireless care and support; my faith-filled friends for their constant prayers; my pastors, Terry, Aaron, and David for their spiritual guidance; and my Christian ladies' LIFE group for their monthly meetings with speakers who shared their stories and prompted me to share my journey.
- To the medical professionals who provided exceptional care and compassion, thank you for your expertise and dedication. Your skill and kindness eased the burdens of my journey.
- Finally, to my faith community, your love, prayers, and fellowship were a constant source of strength and inspiration. Your collective support is a testament to the power of the community in times of need.
- This book is dedicated to all who have walked alongside me, sharing in this challenging, yet transformative journey.

Appendix

This appendix provides additional resources for those seeking further information on cancer, faith-based healing, and spiritual support.

Works Cited

"Coping with Cancer." *National Institute of Health (NIH),* 2019. www.cancer.gov/about-cancercoping. Accessed n.d.

"Getting Beyond. 'Why Me?'"*American Psychological Association (APA).* 2011. www.APA.org. Accessed n.d.

"Mindfulness Meditation." *Association for Psychological Science (APS).* 2019. www.APS.org. Accessed n.d.

"Psychoneuroimmunology." *National Institute of Health (NIH),* 2019. www. newsinhealth.nih.gov. Accessed n.d.

"Sharing Your Story." *National Institute of Health (NIH) Intramural Research Program,* 2025. www.irp.nih.gov. Accessed n.d.

"The Relationship Between Praying and Life Expectancy in Cancer Patients." *Journal of Medicine and Life (JM),* 2015. www.medandlife.org. Accessed n.d.

Williams, Patrick A., et. al. "Supporting Patients with Cancer and Survivors." *American Association for Cancer Research (AACR) Progress Report 2024: Inspiring Science—Fueling Progress—Revolutionizing Care.* 2024. www.AACRJournals.org. Accessed n.d.

List of Support Organizations

American Cancer Society	www.cancer.org
National Cancer Institute	www.cancer.gov
Cancer Care	www.cancercare.org
Check your local area for churches and other organizations that offer cancer support.	

Glossary

This glossary defines some key medical and spiritual terms used throughout the book. They are derived from various sources.

Cancer: A group of diseases characterized by uncontrolled cell growth and the potential to invade and spread to other parts of the body.

Remission: A period when signs and symptoms of a disease, particularly cancer, have diminished or disappeared, though it doesn't necessarily mean the disease is cured.

Spontaneous Remission: The unexpected improvement or cure of a disease, disorder, or illness without the involvement of standard medical treatments.

Faith: A strong belief in God or in the doctrines of a religion, based on spiritual apprehension rather than proof.

Prayer: A solemn request for help or expression of thanks addressed to God or an object of worship.

Meditation: A practice that involves focusing or clearing your mind using a combination of mental and physical techniques.

Divine Intervention: The belief that a higher power, like God, actively and directly intervenes in the affairs of the world often to guide, protect, or alter the course of events.

About the Author

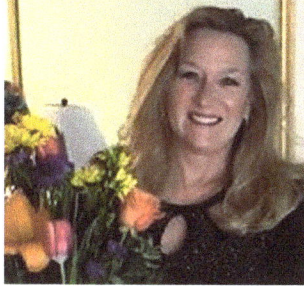

Anne Warren (Van Deventer) Wheeler was an inventor of successful children's products in the '80s and '90s. She appeared several times on national and local news, talk shows, podcasts, and in magazines and newspapers. Later she became a sales and marketing and communications entrepreneur until retirement.

Mrs. Wheeler is a cancer survivor. Diagnosed with cancer in 2022 and 2024, she embarked on a profound journey of faith and healing. Her miraculous recovery and subsequent unexplained remission inspired her to share her personal story of faith, resilience, and the transformative power of belief.

She is an enthusiastic advocate for cancer patients sharing Bella, her mini-goldendoodle, at Coastal Cancer Center. Anne believes in the power of prayer, hope, perseverance, and the enduring strength found in a relationship with God.

Anne and her husband, Bill, reside in Myrtle Beach, South Carolina. Beyond this book, she participates with Bella in Canines for Christ therapy dog ministry, her church community at Ocean View Baptist, and her Del Webb community activities.

Pictures

Left to Right, 1st Row
- Anne's friend and neighbor, Nancie, who was a patient at the Coastal Cancer Center and Bella.
- Anne and Bella (Anne's mini-goldendoodle) at the Coastal Cancer Center

Left to Right, 2nd Row
- Bella's special vest
- Anne, Bella, and Nancie

Left to Right, 3rd Row
- Bella and Nancie
- Bella and Anne

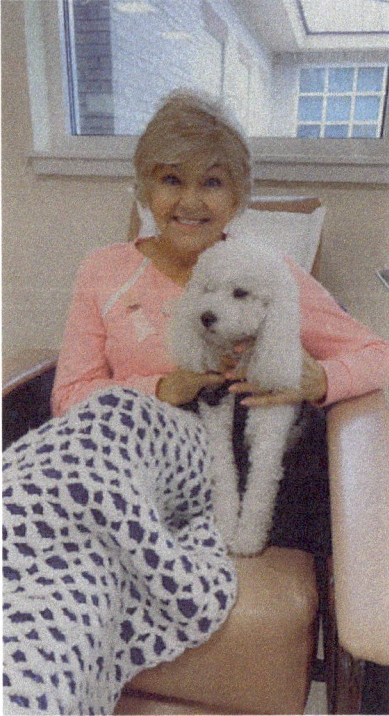
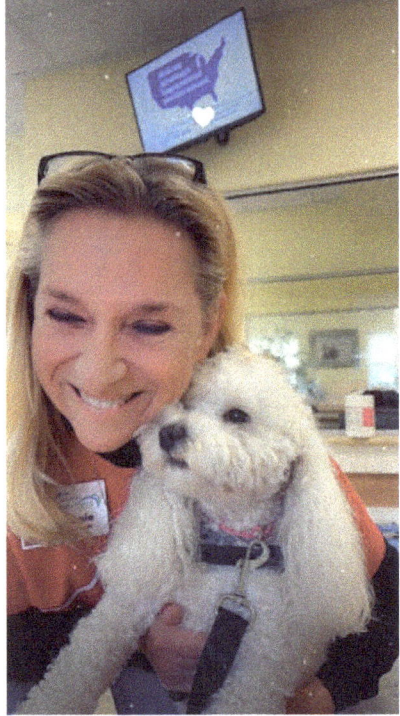
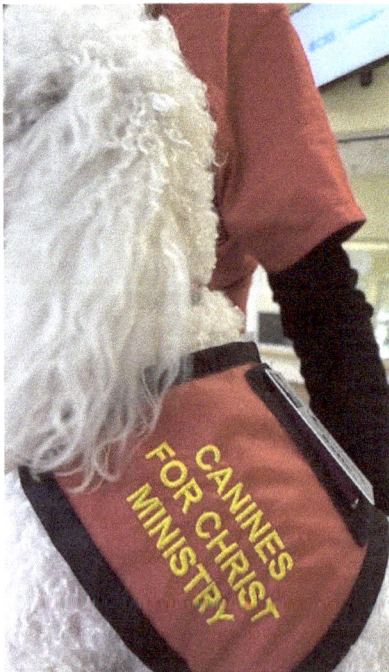
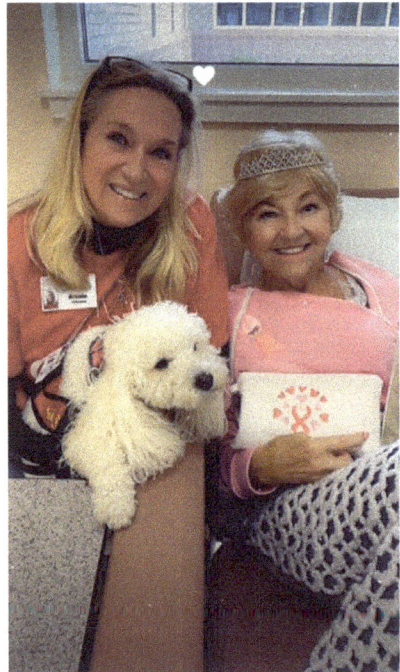

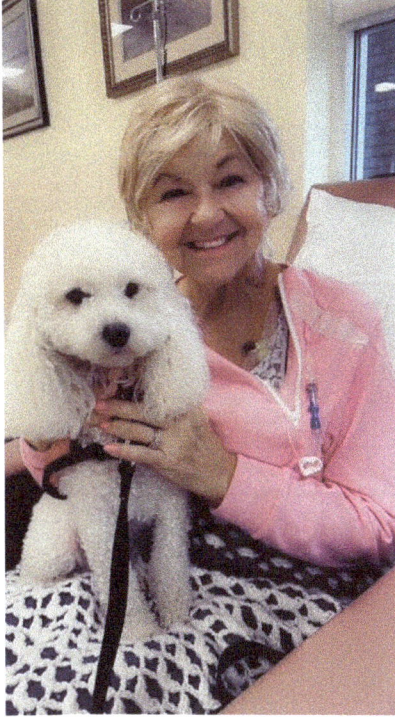
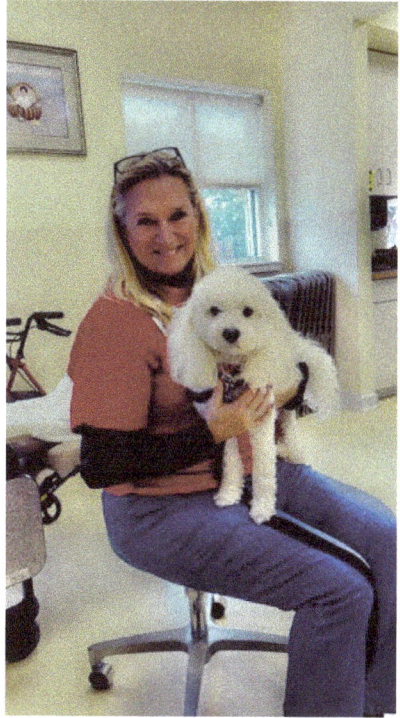

www.ingramcontent.com/pod-product-compliance
Lightning Source LLC
Chambersburg PA
CBHW052024030426
42335CB00026B/3271